THE
TRUTH ABOUT
THYROID

5 Keys to Reverse
Your Thyroid Condition
and Feel Well Again

DISCLAIMER:

THIS BOOK IS FOR EDUCATIONAL
PURPOSES ONLY. THIS BOOK IS NOT
INTENDED AS A SUBSTITUTE FOR THE
MEDICAL ADVICE OF PHYSICIANS. THE
READER SHOULD REGULARLY CONSULT
A PHYSICIAN IN MATTERS RELATING TO
HIS/HER HEALTH AND PARTICULARLY
WITH RESPECT TO ANY SYMPTOMS THAT
MAY REQUIRE DIAGNOSIS OR MEDICAL
ATTENTION. THIS BOOK IS NOT INTENDED
TO DIAGNOSE, CURE, OR TREAT
DISEASE.

ISBN: 9781095432372

Imprint: Independently published

Get the Bonus Resources
That Come with This Book:
http://www.ThyroidHealthInfo.com/
Book-Bonuses

Dedication

This book is dedicated to my clients who, for over 27 years, have trusted me in guiding them on the path of optimum health.

Your willingness, desire, and teachability to get well, combined with my system, has created the best conditions for transforming your body, mind, and feeling vibrant again.

Thank you for your commitment to your highest and best health. Seeing your results come to life fuels my motivation to continue helping champions like you.

You and your family deserve full, happy, healthy and vibrant lives!

Table of Contents

Introduction

The purpose of this book is to help you **understand how your thyroid truly works** and give you the information you need to take back control of your health.

The reason thyroid symptoms are often misunderstood and misdiagnosed is their *complexity*. The thyroid is involved in <u>ALL</u> physiological processes in the body; every cell requires thyroid hormone to function properly.

Thyroid conditions are often treated in very limited ways—the focus is on using medication to adjust TSH (thyroid stimulating hormone) to 'normal' levels. But thyroid problems involve much, much more.

Your thyroid condition may affect your reproductive system, immune system, nervous system and digestive system, and that's not all. In the vast majority of cases, thyroid issues are the result of an autoimmune condition known as Hashimoto's disease. This condition is rarely tested in conventional medicine, and almost never addressed in a meaningful way if it is diagnosed. Yet with proper support, Hashimoto's disease, and the thyroid problems it causes, can be well managed. Often symptoms are minimized or even completely resolved.

I am under the firm belief (based on proof I share with you in this book) that with the right support you can almost certainly reverse your metabolic imbalances and feel amazing.

A comprehensive approach to the complexity of your thyroid condition can sort out and guide therapeutic support that is targeted, safe and effective.

Modifications that involve exercise, diet, stress management and other lifestyle choices can restore balance and correct dysfunction throughout the body in specific ways. You'll feel better because your body recovers and heals, and you'll have solutions that can help you long term.

Medication for symptom management is all most doctors have to offer their patients with thyroid conditions because that is what they're taught in medical school. Sometimes damage to the thyroid or other circumstances make thyroid medication necessary. In cases like these, addressing the underlying cause of the patient's condition often makes a tremendous difference in how well the medicine works and in how the patient feels.

It may be possible to reduce the amount of medication your body requires to function effectively once you've recovered optimal health through holistic support. If you'd like to get to the bottom of *why* you feel the way you do, this book can help you. Together, we can make lasting improvements in your health and quality of life. I am sharing the method that allowed me to reclaim my own health. This is a process that was born out of frustration with the conventional system that did not provide me the answers I was seeking.

At 38 I found myself having severe fatigue to the point of it being nearly impossible to get up in the mornings. I was gaining weight out of control. I felt irritable and exhausted. It was virtually impossible to lose weight. I had aches and pains in the soles of my feet and muscles. I was losing my hair (which was disheartening). I had brain fog, mood swings, and I felt as if I was 80 years old!

Had I been to a rheumatologist I would have been diagnosed with fibromyalgia. Had I been to a podiatrist I would have been diagnosed with plantar fasciitis. Had I been to a psychiatrist I would have been diagnosed with an emotional disorder. I was sick and tired of feeling sick and tired and I had no idea what was happening to my system. I needed to find a solution.

I was so tired that once my husband had to carry me to the car to take a vacation. All my tests were "normal." My well-meaning colleague suggested antidepressants. I knew that I did not have a deficiency of antidepressants. I had never had depression in my life. There was only one solution: I was going to have to figure it out on my own.

After spending a fortune on my medical training, I spent another fortune to find answers. I aligned myself with like-minded mentors and became a student. I rearranged my schedule to work three days a week, embarking on my own "heal thyself journey" while still helping others as a physician.

One of the most vulnerable and scary discoveries I made on that journey is this...

GETTING WELL IS NOT COVERED BY INSURANCE!

Meaning, the care covered by my personal insurance would NOT help *me* transform my health. Also, that same insurance-based methodology was limiting my ability to help my *clients*.

Can you understand how conflicting and painful that felt?

The knowledge was eating at me.

I was already looking into alternative ways to get the help I needed. One of my mentors, an acupuncturist,

Johanne Rose, sat in my office and waited hours for me to finish working with patients. She sat me down and said, "Hilda, you need to stop. You're trying to help people in a holistic way, but you're confined by insurance-based limitations, and it's affecting your health."

That was the day I chose to transform from "insurance-based primary-care" to a "consulting-only non-insurance-based" practice.

You know what? I've helped hundreds more people – potentially keeping them on earth longer, living full, healthy, vibrant lives with their loved ones letting go of ineffective and antiquated methodologies.

I discovered my answers in an unconventional way and I cracked the code, turning myself around without band aid prescription medications or surgical procedures.

I successfully *reset* my health path, *reversed* my underlying metabolic and nutritional imbalances and *reclaimed* my health and my life.

The result: Vibrant transformation, energy, mental clarity and permanent weight and belly fat loss. I feel and look 10-15 years-younger, people ask me if I have had "work" done. I feel vibrant and have been able to flourish my career and empower many people like you. So, I am here to support you. If you are "stuck" and have done everything you know to do, and you are still struggling with fatigue, brain fog, weight gain, and decreased sense of well-being, **it is not your fault.**

I am here to give you a glimpse of hope and I have made it my life's work to decode the process. I will transfer to you what I have learned, saving you a ten to fifteen-year learning curve. I want to make it clear that knowledge is only wisdom when paired with action.

You owe it to yourself to live in your best, most vibrant body and mind! to go from health "in default" to health "by design," full of vitality, energy and focus.

BEFORE   AFTER

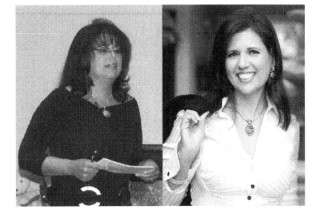

Who is This Book For?

I once heard a story about a man walking with his granddaughter on a beach. They came across thousands of starfish washed up on the sand after a storm went through the night before.

The starfish were baking and dying in the sun, and the grandfather began picking up one starfish at a time. He bent down slowly, grabbed a starfish, walked it to the water's edge, and threw it back into the sea.

After five starfish, the grand-daughter started complaining...

"Poppa, this is taking sooO long! There are thooouusands of starfish. What difference does this make?"

The grandfather held up one starfish and replied...

"For this one, it makes <u>ALL</u> the difference in the world."

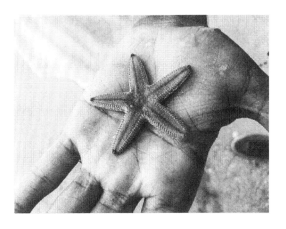

This book could make *all* the difference for YOU if you are between 35 and 60 years of age, live a busy and productive life, and value your health.

... For you who have been feeling out of sorts with your energy and have not been able to find answers, but in every physical exam you are told that "all" your tests are normal.

... For you who take thyroid replacement but still feel hypothyroid symptoms, frustrated with stubborn belly fat, feeling tired and would like to say good-bye to brain fog.

... For you who have done everything to try and solve your health challenges but are still stuck.

Common Symptoms to Overcome

Many women reach a point where they do not feel the way they used to. It may be in their late 30s or 40s, or later in life when they realize that physically, mentally and emotionally, they're struggling. Health issues that start out small may seem to snowball, or signs of a problem that's overwhelming, may very quickly set in.

- Mental sharpness slips. It's difficult to concentrate. Brain fog slows you down.

- You have trouble falling asleep or you wake up too early, and it's difficult to drag yourself out of bed.

- You're so tired after work, you stop socializing; chores like food shopping and laundry, become major ordeals due to exhaustion.

- The enthusiasm and passion for life you may have known has been replaced by a much bleaker, pessimistic view.

- You can't seem to shed a pound of extra weight you've gained, especially in the belly area, no matter how little you eat or how much you exercise.

- You're taking over-the-counter remedies and pills for achy joints and muscles or headaches.

- You've almost given up believing you'll ever be physically fit or feel like your old self again.

- You assume or been told by a health-care provider that your experiencing is "normal" and just a part of aging. *(This one is so common, and makes me so upset to hear because it is NOT TRUE!).*

- You may have had your thyroid tested and been told that it's fine. Thyroid symptoms are often compounded with sex hormone-related changes.

If you've ever wished there was something more that could be done—a real solution— I have great news.

There is hope!

No matter how long you've struggled, how many doctors you've seen or how many medications you've tried, it <u>is absolutely possible</u> for you to feel much better. You can lose the extra weight— even the stubborn belly fat. You can get a great night's sleep. You can wake up refreshed. You can regain your energy and it will carry you through the day and last through the evening.

One of the most common scenarios I see in my practice is a 38-year-old female who cannot lose weight.

Her abdomen is bloating after meals. She's constipated and tired all the time. When she exercises, she gets pain all over her body, and feels worse. She has done many diets and loses weight only to gain it back again.

Now she cannot lose the weight even if she starves herself. Her weight gain is 'even' throughout her whole body. The bottom of her feet hurt when she gets out of bed. Has been told everything is normal during her physical. She is starting to feel hopeless.

She wonders: "is this is how it's going to be for the rest of my life?"

She keeps going to keep up with the demands of her life. Her tiredness is worse if she sits down. She drinks caffeine and eats sugar to make it through the day. She's still exhausted. She has her thyroid tested, but she only receives one test: a TSH. She is told the TSH is high normal. Her doctor says, "we will watch it". She insists that something is wrong. She needs to know her *Metabolic Profile* (more on this later) and have specialized tests completed – which are not normally done as part of her routine physical – to get to the root of the situation. *Most commonly she'll discover that her symptoms relate to much more than "just" her thyroid.*

Once all the dots are connected, based on her individual metabolic markers, and the *5 Keys of Activation* are applied in the specific order to meet her needs, *she* will turn around and her condition will too.

Three Stages: Your Journey to a Full Solution

In my experience there are three stages people go through when it comes to thyroid related issues.

The first stage is when the person suspects that they have a thyroid dysfunction. They're starting to see symptoms, and do initial research, yet haven't started a plan of action.

The second stage is the person that went to see the doctor, yet have been told their test results are fine.

The third stage is the person who has already been under the care of a physician. They've been diagnosed with either hypothyroidism or Hashimoto's thyroiditis. They may have been given a prescription medication. After a while on the thyroid replacement they are still not feeling optimal. They may be told that their tests are normal on current dose of replacement. Yet, their symptoms continue.

Over the following pages, I will talk with you about each stage. As you read on, ask yourself which stage you fit within.

YOU HAVE SYMPTOMS, YET HAVEN'T CREATED A PLAN OF ACTION

You may be feeling sluggish, frustrated with weight gain and forgetful. You start talking to your friends, Dr. Google, and Dr. Facebook.

Suddenly you realize that you have many other symptoms that could be associated with low thyroid.

You decide to take matters into your own hands and read books, articles and blogs and end up quite confused. You may try natural remedies and supplements. Things don't get better and you decide to see a doctor.

YOU'VE SEEN A DOCTOR, THEY'RE SAYING EVERYTHING'S NORMAL

This is when the frustration starts building up. You have looked at every symptom of low thyroid and you have most of them. You are convinced that something will show when you visit your primary care doctor.

But your tests are all normal.

Oh boy! I can relate.

There are three things to be aware of at this stage.

1. Most doctors <u>only</u> do a TSH test. I find that this is not enough to show the entire picture.

2. The second thing to be aware of, is that most doctors <u>do not</u> test for nutritional deficiencies that can affect thyroid function.

3. Lastly, normal results are based on averages of the population and the ranges are too wide. A test can be normal but that does not mean it is *optimal or* useful for making a plan.

You've Been Diagnosed with Low Thyroid, Given Replacement, But Are Still Having Symptoms

After a while your symptoms have progressed and you request another set of tests. Now the low thyroid shows on the tests and your doctor offers you thyroid replacement. You start the replacement, yet the changes are incremental at best. Meaning, you feel about 50 percent improvement since you have been taking replacement, but there are still lingering symptoms.

At this point, you may start feeling somewhat hopeless. Also, you may have been made to feel as if it's all in your head.

There are five things to consider...

1. You may be taking the wrong type of prescription <u>for you</u>.

2. You may be taking other prescriptions that are interfering with your replacement.

3. You may have nutritional deficiencies of key nutrients needed for optimal thyroid function.

4. Your thyroid dysfunction may have an underlying autoimmune component that has not been addressed.

5. You are taking the correct type of replacement for you but were never provided the correct directions on how to take it.

... Or a combination of the above.

NO MATTER WHICH STAGE YOU'RE IN...

If you have desire to get well, you're willing to make simple changes, and you're teachable: you are in the greatest position to transform your health through a set of five principles I coined, called...

The 5 Keys of Activation

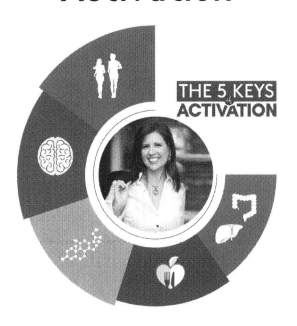

Visit: http://www.ThyroidHealthInfo.com/Book-Bonuses
for bonus material that comes with the book.

The *5 Keys of Activation* may seem familiar to you. You may have tried addressing them individually, but perhaps never looked at all of them at the same time. In my experience serving people like you, the Five Keys are the factors that (combined) have the biggest impact on your health. They all influence each other, either positively or negatively. Understanding these keys and unlocking their imbalances will empower you to enjoy vibrant health for life.

Have you ever tried to solve a Rubik's cube? Helping you turn around your imbalances is like solving an individualized Rubik's cube. Each key is important, but the order of unlocking the imbalances need to be unique to you. Some people need to address gastrointestinal health first. Other people may need to address Nutrition, or Hormone Balance first.

The ORDER the *5 Keys of Activation* are Applied Can Make or Break the RESULTS you get!

Following my method, *the Five Keys of Activation*, has allowed me to help my clients decrease belly fat, achieve more energy, increase their mental focus, enjoy better sleep, and develop a stronger immune system.

KEY #1: GASTROINTESTINAL AND LIVER HEALTH

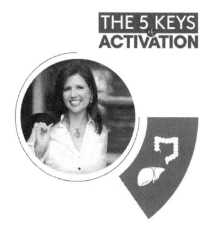

Gut health and liver health take center stage when it comes to overall health.

Seventy percent of your immune system interactions happen in your gut, the gut immune system gets formed during breast-feeding as babies.

Most people with chronic disease, autoimmune conditions and inflammatory chronic disease have an underlying gut imbalance.

You do not need to live with bowel cramps, bloating, chronic constipation and loose stools. (It amazes me when a client thinks it's *normal* to have bowel movements *once or twice* weekly. That is NOT normal). These are symptoms of gut inflammation. Most people with those type of symptoms are told they have IBS

(Irritable Bowel Syndrome) and are dismissed by the conventional wisdom.

When dealing with bloating after meals is important to know if it is mainly upper or lower abdominal bloating as that simple distinction will likely determine the course of action.

Our Gut barrier is only one cell layer thick. The cells in the lining are meant to be tightly adjacent to one another to avoid unwanted particles to go from the intestine into the bloodstream. When the tight junctions between the cells become disrupted (Leaky-Gut) it's like the "caulking" is gone and now there is passage of unwanted particles into the bloodstream. These particles get identified by a series of lymph nodes that sit in what is called the "retroperitoneum," just a fancy name for saying "behind the intestines". An autoimmune response gets triggered that can result in food sensitivities or autoimmune conditions.

When gut inflammation crosses the gut barrier into the bloodstream, it can also reach and cross the blood brain barrier and show up as brain inflammation symptoms. The Gut-Brain connection is important in helping get to the root cause of brain fog.

Here are some factors that can trigger leaky gut and gut inflammation: Stress, inflammatory foods, alcohol, multiple antibiotic use, prescription and OTC medications. I know you do not want to hear this, but the most common inflammatory foods include: sugar, coffee, gluten, dairy, peanuts, soy, corn, shellfish, eggs and tomatoes. Though it may help get rid of some symptoms, just because you avoid inflammatory foods it does not mean you will properly repair your gut lining. In addition, if you are having sugar and carbohydrate cravings, we need to deal with that before you embark on a quest of stopping sugar, or you may fail in your attempt and become frustrated again.

The liver is more than a filtration organ. It is involved in hormone regulation, cholesterol and triglyceride metabolism, glucose stores and inflammatory markers production. For example, the conversion to the active form of thyroid occurs primarily in the liver and gastrointestinal tract.

Many people make the crucial mistake to engage in "liver detox" programs without first making sure they have repaired their gut lining. It's as if you put Drano® in your sink but your pipes have holes. Would you ever do that? Of course not, you would repair the pipe first. Releasing toxins into a broken GI (Gastrointestinal) tract will cause more damage than good. It can result in tiredness, fatigue, brain fog, headaches, body aches and rashes.

Another problem with the "so called" detox programs is that they often use products that create an imbalance between what is known as Phase I and Phase II detoxification in the liver. This leads to the person getting headaches and "flu-like symptoms".

Many times, people are told this is part of a "healing crisis".

Please know there is not such a thing as a "healing crisis." If your body is screaming, there is a reason.

If you have had your gallbladder removed, you may experience chronic gastrointestinal symptoms such as loose stools or diarrhea, especially if you eat a fatty meal.

Summary: Your GI tract and Liver play a significant role in your thyroid health. There are specific nutrients that can aid in repairing the gut.

Next, we'll look at the second *Key of Activation*: nutrition.

KEY #2:
NUTRITION

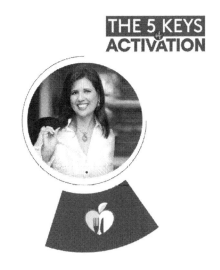

Selenium, B-Vitamins, Iron, Iodine and Zinc are important as it relates to thyroid function.

Proper absorption of nutrients from food and supplements requires a healthy gut lining. As discussed above, consumption of inflammatory foods promotes gastrointestinal inflammation, which can interfere with nutrient absorption.

When looking at nutrition it is important to look at two areas, food consumption (macronutrients) and supplementation (micronutrients).

Most of the foods we eat are depleted of key nutrients because the soil in which the food is grown is deprived of key minerals.

Micronutrient deficiencies are often at the root of metabolic imbalances. Micronutrients also help your body properly process toxic exposures.

If you are having sugar or salt cravings it is likely your body needs to replenish something else. Once you provide your body what it needs, your sugar cravings will stop.

Most people decide they need to change how they eat. They start with diets. They rely on their will-power, which inevitably fades at some point. What if, we could correct your imbalances based on your individual needs and suddenly you don't crave the sugar?

Supplements are only as good as the foods you eat. To use supplements, without specifically knowing which nutrients you need, lends itself to what I call "green medicine." Meaning, you start using a different supplement for every symptom or condition. That is a problem because using supplements this way does not address the root cause. You may be taking something you don't need, and may need something else.

Vitamins (vital-amines) and minerals are important cofactors for many normal physiologic and enzymatic reactions. Not all supplements are created equal, there is variability in quality. After over twenty-five years of incorporating supplement support, I choose to only use high quality formulas that work. The most expensive supplement is the one that does not work. As one of my clients likes to say, "the proof is in the pudding."

Summary: Nutrition also plays a significant role in your thyroid health. Finding out exactly what your body needs takes the guesswork away from your plan of action. Not everyone needs A-Z supplementation.

Next, we'll look at the third *Key of Activation*: hormones.

KEY #3:
HORMONES

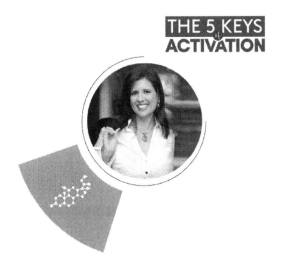

THE 5 KEYS ACTIVATION

Our bodies have many hormones naturally. Everything about your being – what you look like, your mindset, your stamina, and whether you lose or gain fat – is directly tied to your hormone balance. Specific hormone imbalances create specific body shapes. Hormones do not work in isolation; they form an intricate network. Hormones decline as we age, and we age when our hormones decline. Healthy hormone metabolism depends on a healthy gut and a healthy liver. Micronutrient deficiencies can interfere with proper hormone metabolism. Hormone imbalances are often at the root cause of difficulty losing weight and fat loss resistance despite adequate exercise. Hormone imbalances can contribute to inflammation. Hormone imbalances are often at the root cause of neurotransmitter imbalances. I look at the entire hormonal picture: sex hormones (estrogen, progesterone, testosterone, and sex hormone binding globulin), thyroid hormones, adrenal hormones and blood sugar regulation & weight loss resistance hormones. Thyroid Hormones are of utmost importance. That is why I am expanding on them in this book.

*** Just a quick note: the following part on Thyroid Hormones is technical in nature. I included this part in the book for the people who want to learn more about the specific science behind their thyroid. In addition, you'll learn which parts of our bodies produce hormones. If any of the following is confusing, consider visiting the bonus materials in this book. I created a video that deconstructs this topic using clear visuals. You'll love it.

THYROID HORMONES

There are two main types of thyroid imbalances, high and low thyroid.

High thyroid function is known as hyperthyroidism and it requires the immediate attention of a conventional endocrinologist. Symptoms of high thyroid include, palpitations, feeling agitated, jittery or diarrhea. If the reason for the high thyroid symptoms is too much thyroid replacement, it is simply a matter of decreasing the dose.

Low thyroid function is known as hypothyroidism and is usually associated with:

- Fatigue that gets worse if you sit
- Brain fog
- Hair loss
- Coarse, dry hair

- Dry Skin
- Feeling "thick"
- Weight gain
- Swollen round facial features
- Lateral third eyebrow loss
- Constipation
- Joint aches
- Cold intolerance
- Muscle cramps
- Irregular periods
- Infertility
- Plantar foot pain
- Overall lack of wellbeing
- Palpitations

When thyroid is low it puts undue stress on your brain, your heart and your adrenal glands.

Here is an overview of how the thyroid system works. If everything is working the way it is intended to, the brain produces TSH which goes to the thyroid gland and stimulates the production of T4. Then T4 takes a tour in the bloodstream and gets to the liver where it converts to T3. Our cells only have receptors for T3. When T3 finds the cell receptors that sit on the cell walls it moves inside the cells to produce energy. (See diagram on next page).

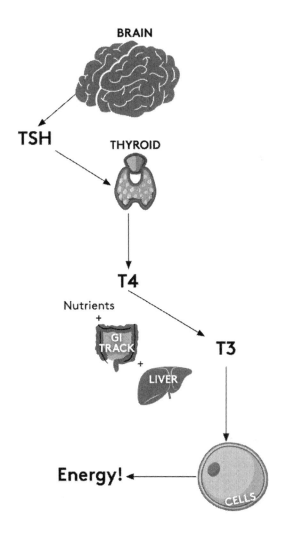

THYROID HORMONE #1: TSH

TSH stands for "Thyroid Stimulating Hormone".

TSH is often considered the main thyroid hormone for diagnosing hypo- or hyperthyroidism. TSH levels are high when thyroid function is low (hypothyroidism). Conversely, low TSH means an overactive thyroid (hyperthyroidism).

TSH is released by a gland in the brain (pituitary gland) to increase thyroid function by increasing T4 at the thyroid gland level (see diagram above).

Unfortunately, conventional endocrinologists and other conventional practitioners often do not look beyond a TSH. However, I prefer to do more than just a TSH test. A TSH by itself may not uncover the entire picture on people with persistent low thyroid symptoms. It takes more than a TSH to get to the root cause of a low thyroid. I have a functional endocrinology and holistic mindset and I transfer that to my clients by looking at multiple markers.

A "normal" TSH is not the same as an ideal TSH. The normal ranges are too wide in their scope.

THYROID HORMONE #2: FREE T4

Considered a precursor hormone, T4 is converted into T3 as required by cells throughout the body. Generally, this conversion of T4 to T3 occurs outside the thyroid gland, typically in the liver and gastrointestinal tract.

Although T4 is more abundant in the blood than T3, it is much less potent. This is important to understand why you can be receiving thyroid replacement and still feel hypothyroid.

THYROID HORMONE #3: FREE T3

Free T3 is the main thyroid hormone in terms of biological activity that regulates metabolism and growth throughout the body. It is more potent than T4 and directly affects the heart, blood vessels, bone, muscle and brain. T3 increases a person's metabolic rate, controls body temperature, regulates neurotransmitter synthesis (mood), impacts heart rate and oversees the conversion of food into energy. Our cells only have receptors for T3, therefore the conversion of T4 to T3 is paramount for proper optimal metabolism.

Certain nutritional deficiencies, stress and some prescription medications such as oral estrogens, oral contraceptives, and beta blockers will interfere with the conversion of T4 to T3. Micronutrients that are needed for T4 to convert to T3 include Iodine, Selenium, B vitamins, Iron, and Zinc. If your free T3 is low you will have low thyroid symptoms even if your TSH and T4 are within acceptable limits.

THYROID HORMONE #4: REVERSE T3

Reverse T3 opposes the biological action of T3. It slows metabolism and renders T3 in the body biologically inactive. The rate of rT3 production relative to T3 will increase in times of stress (high cortisol) and in the presence of nutrient deficiencies, inflammation or certain medications.

In addition, people that do unhealthy weight loss with caloric restrictions and yo-yo dieting tend to have elevated levels of Reverse T3. In essence, reverse T3 blocks the activity of T3.

ADDITIONAL THYROID MARKERS:

Anti-TPO (Antibodies to Thyroid Peroxidase).

Thyroid Peroxidase (TPO) is an enzyme that initiates the formation of T4. Antibodies to TPO indicate autoimmunity where the body is attacking TPO. People with anti-TPO have a higher chance of developing hypothyroidism than those who do not have antibodies to TPO. The presence of anti-thyroid peroxidase antibodies is otherwise known as Hashimoto's Thyroiditis.

A WORD ABOUT HASHIMOTO'S THYROIDITIS:

Hashimoto's Thyroiditis is the most common cause of hypothyroidism in developed countries. It is an autoimmune condition. This is important because most people with Hashimoto's are told they have a thyroid condition and there is not much they can do about controlling the antibodies.

Since seventy percent of our immune system is driven by our gut, gut health is very important for Hashimoto's management. I have seen clients have significant improvements in TPO titers by addressing gut health. Depending on the severity of gut inflammation and the length of time that it has gone unchecked, addressing gut health may be a complex process. Avoiding gluten is *only part* of the solution, usually the gut lining is in need of deeper repair and the inflammation needs to be addressed.

In my experience, it is impossible to successfully address Hashimoto's without addressing the gut-liver connection, toxic exposures, nutritional deficiencies, food sensitivities and environmental factors. These connections are not addressed when you see a conventional doctor and the only solution typically offered is thyroid replacement.

Over the years, I have met many people that have already been looking for a holistic solution to Hashimoto's and have done various versions of the components I discussed above without significant results. Then, when we customize the *5 Keys of Activation* for them, address imbalances for their unique situation, they turn around.

It's common for people with Hashimoto's to have a goiter or enlarged thyroid in addition to multiple benign nodules. If you are ever told you have a thyroid nodule that is growing, or close to one centimeter in length, you need to seek the attention of an endocrinologist that can help you decide if it should be removed and looked at to make sure it's not thyroid cancer.

WHAT ABOUT THYROID REPLACEMENT?

Thyroid is one of the most important hormones in our body. It affects everything and anything you can think of. Over the years, I have seen people who need thyroid replacement get a prescription by their doctor refuse to take it. On the other hand, I have seen people that clearly need thyroid replacement be denied replacement by their doctor under the premise their results are "only borderline." I have also seen people taking the prescription, with "normal tests" still feeling completely hypothyroid.

There seems to be a tremendous amount of misinformation and confusion when it comes to thyroid replacement. The answers are not always straightforward, hence the importance for **individualization**.

The conventional way of replacing thyroid is using only synthetic T4 replacement. There are many people that don't feel full relief using synthetic T4 by itself. These people benefit from a combination of T4 and T3. The most common form of prescription T3 is synthetic and only stays in the body for about four hours, which does not help.

There are options for T4 and T3 replacement using glandular extract but most conventional doctors have not been trained to use them. Glandular thyroid is manufactured by a pharmaceutical company and must keep industry standards of purity and potency. Many people do well on these types of products. When choosing a glandular I prefer Nature Throid® or Westhroid®, when appropriate.

In my experience, most people that are *only* given synthetic T4 to address their thyroid feel partial relief and still complain of low thyroid symptoms. **The best way to address thyroid health is by following a comprehensive and holistic approach.** Unfortunately, some people think that "holistic" means "without thyroid replacement." That is not the case.

Holistic means:

"Taking in the 'whole' picture and basing your choices upon *complete* information."

Regardless of the type of replacement you use, it is important that it is taken in the morning, on an empty stomach by itself. You'll want to wait a minimum of 30-60 minutes to eat or drink anything other than water. You should not take supplements or other prescription medications within that time either. I personally don't like to consider thyroid replacement as a true prescription medication. We were born with thyroid in our body and not replacing it when you clearly need it leaves your body at risk for a sluggish metabolism and chronic disease.

In the case of Hashimoto's thyroiditis, if caught early it is possible to avoid thyroid replacement. Some people have been hypothyroid for so long that it puts unnecessary stress on the adrenal glands. If you need to take thyroid replacement, but you are not able to tolerate it even at low doses, chances are that your adrenal glands need support.

THYROID HORMONES TAKEAWAYS:

- TSH is produced in the brain.

- TSH signals the thyroid gland to produce T4.

- T4 tours through the body, and as it passes the liver, converts to T3.

- T3 goes around the bloodstream and gets to work in the form of Free T3.

- Our cells only have receptors for T3.

- T3 goes inside the cells and aids in energy reactions.

- The conversion of T4 to T3 can be affected by nutritional deficiencies, stress and prescription medications.

- When testing T4 and T3 you want the "free" hormone.

- Thyroid hormone is essential for optimal health.

- Do not ignore the need for thyroid replacement.

- A TSH test can be normal and you can still feel hypothyroid symptoms.

- A comprehensive approach is often needed in the presence of Hypothyroidism with or without Hashimoto's Thyroiditis.

Summary: Hormones play a significant role in your health and thyroid is one of those hormones. Getting a clear understanding of your hormones empowers us to make the most informed and intelligent choice about what plan of action to take.

Next, we'll look at the fourth *Key of Activation*: Neurotransmitter Balance.

KEY #4:
NEUROTRANSMITTER
BALANCE

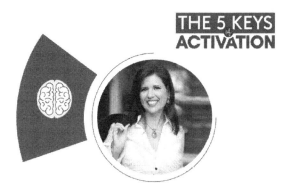

Neurotransmitters are the chemicals that send signals through our brain cells.

There is a relationship between neurotransmitters, the nervous system and hormones referred to as the "Neuro-endocrine Connection." There is also a relationship between neurotransmitters and the gut referred to as the "Gut-Brain Connection."

Neurotransmitter imbalances are associated with chronic external stress, gut inflammation, nutritional deficiencies, hormone imbalances, internal stress, head trauma and environmental-toxic exposures.

Movement and exercise are well-established ways of supporting neurotransmitter balance. There are individuals that will over exercise even when their body is "running on empty" as a form of self-medication through endorphins.

Summary: Neurotransmitter health affects mindset, motivation and the quality of your thinking. Thyroid health affects the functions of your brain.

Next, we'll look at the fifth and last *Key of Activation*: Movement.

KEY #5:
MOVEMENT

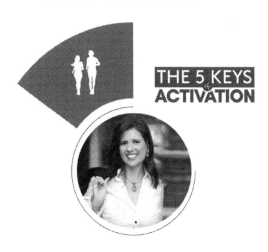

As we age, our bodies tend to lose muscle and gain fat, this is known as sarcopenia. Preserving your muscle is important for proper metabolism.

What is the point of losing weight if you lose muscle in the process? Many people that do drastic diets lose muscle mass and gain more fat. This is the Yo-Yo effect.

Consider this for a moment: the best way to lose fat is to "fill your tank of fuel" first. That means that by the time you introduce exercise you have already started correcting imbalances and decreasing inflammation.

You have gained some energy physically, mentally and emotionally. You are ready to exercise and get the results that you desperately want. You start seeing results with less overall effort on your part when you do it that way.

I know first-hand what it is to feel terrible "flu like" symptoms and swollen lymph glands after exercise. I know what it feels like to have a well-meaning trainer push you when your body is saying "please stop! the tank needs to get filled with fuel!" It's about working smarter not harder, and being able to see the results you have not been able to achieve before.

Resistance-training exercise is key to preserve bone and muscle.

When your thyroid hormones are not optimal, it's as if you are running with an "empty tank." Trying to exercise this way may be a painful and frustrating experience.

SUMMARY OF
THE *5 KEYS OF ACTIVATION*

Again, the *5 Keys of Activation* are:

1. Gastrointestinal and Liver Health
2. Nutrition
3. Hormones
4. Neurotransmitter Balance
5. Movement

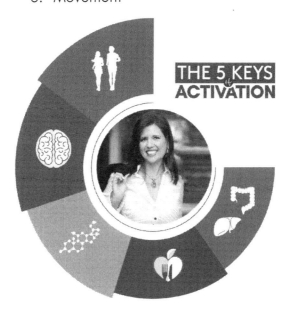

The *5 Keys of Activation* work like a "matrix." They are five independent parts that are interrelated with each other.

Looking at the human body this way has allowed me to move from seeing the body's systems as "islands," and instead viewing them as one world. This leads me to one of the most profound revelations I've had about the human body, health, and vibrant living...

WHERE DISEASE STARTS

Disease doesn't "just happen" overnight; it is an evolution. When someone gets a disease diagnosis, that disease is the *result* of imbalances happening over time.

There are phases that occur before the physical expression of disease. These phases can work both ways: a downward descending spiral into poor health and premature death, or an upward ascension into ideal health, vibrancy, and youthfulness.

Here are the phases...

THE CELLULAR PHASE

Our cells are equipped to host complex internal biochemical reactions. They need enzymes, nutrients, and co-factors to be present and work effectively to create energy production.

Think of this phase like a new car. If you fill it with the right fuel and clean it regularly, you'll maintain its value longer and keep it running efficiently. Most people run their body as if there are no consequences to their actions, like driving a car with unlimited mileage, zero maintenance, and zero fueling.

THE BIOCHEMICAL BLOOD ABNORMALITIES PHASE

At this stage there may be symptoms that come and go, or no symptoms at all.

This stage reminds me of a tale of a couple and their dog.

Bob and Anne are sitting on their front porch with their dog, Lady. Lady is howling in pain. Anne says, "Why's Lady howling?" Bob replies, "Oh, she's sitting on a nail." Anne says, "Why doesn't she get up?"

Bob responds:

"Well, honey, I guess it just doesn't hurt *that* much."

Sometimes our pain isn't painful *enough* to get up and do something about it. We tolerate it, ignore it, and justify it; trying to sweep it under the rug and hope it will go away. Yet, what's happening beneath the veil is compounding into something worse. Ironically, the *Biochemical Blood Abnormalities Phase* is a great window of opportunity to identify and reverse metabolic imbalances and potentially avoid chronic disease.

THE SUFFERING DISEASE PHASE

Debilitating symptoms ensue. You can't work efficiently and earn money due to zero energy, massive weight gain, inability to think, out of control mood swings, aching pains in your body, etc.

By the time you reach this level you have already been living with advanced biochemical blood test abnormalities and cellular imbalances for quite some time, and now it's finally caught up to you.

It's unfortunate that most people reach this stage, and in most cases their disease was potentially reversible if they had the right information. Then, they get caught up in the vortex of conventional over-prescription and more side effects.

You have to make a conscious decision to reset your path in order to get off this hamster wheel.

Ignoring the body's attempts to scream at you for help and not taking the time to clearly identify the root cause of malfunctions is a sure path to chronic disease.

If you're ready to embrace a whole new world of energy, bodyweight, mental clarity, and sense of well-being in life, you have to ask yourself an important question:

"At what phase will I take action?"

Remember you only get one body and it becomes your place of residence for the rest of your life.

Final Thoughts

I wrote this book to help you understand how your body works in regard to your thyroid. I designed this book to give you the information you need to take control of your health.

Your thyroid is involved in ALL physiological processes in your body; every cell requires thyroid hormone to function properly. It's important to remember your thyroid symptoms are linked to the *5 Keys of Activation.*

The best way to get the most effective plan is by analyzing all five for your body.

WHAT TO DO NEXT

If you visit:

http://www.ThyroidHealthInfo.com/ Book-Bonuses

You can get access to a series of special bonuses that relate to thyroid health and *the 5 Keys of Activation*.

If you are serious about achieving optimal health and potentially avoiding chronic disease, you'll LOVE the material my team and I have put together for you.

Thank you

I am so very thankful you discovered this book. I hope you found the information useful, and please stay in contact. I have so much more for you on the topic of thyroid, hormones, health and wellbeing. You have the power to transform your life.

It's my greatest wish for you to see that new possibility for yourself.

Sincerely,

Dr. Hilda

About the Author

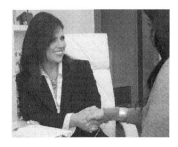

Dr. Hilda Maldonado, M.D. is a practicing medical doctor who has bridged the gap between conventional, alternative and anti-aging medicine. She has helped many people attain optimum health through her unique blend of treatment modalities.

She has completed an advanced postdoctoral fellowship in anti-aging and regenerative medicine. Her practice is located in Westlake Village, CA where she resides with her supportive family.

Besides staying busy with her family, friends, church and practice, Doctor Maldonado is a horse enthusiast. She enjoys going on trail rides and learning horsemanship skills.